# ATKINS DIET

How to Obtain Your Ideal
Weight with the Most Popular
Low Carb Diet Worldwide

By ERIK FISHNER

# Table of Contents

# Introduction

Following a low-carb diet could be a satisfying experience for those who want to lose weight. People who have a problem with lack of satisfaction and hunger while following a certain type of diet have discovered that low carb diet seems to be the answer to this struggle. All of a sudden, all your cravings disappear, your fat fades away, and you'll feel a lot better.

Unfortunately, that's not the case for everyone. There are people who follow low carb diet and still have problems with losing weight. They are following the plan impeccably, and perhaps the cravings go away, and they even follow a workout routine, but just can't seem to lose weight no matter what they do. That is where the Atkins diet comes into the picture. This form of diet was developed for people who follow the low-carb diet but can't make any difference on their weight.

Since the introduction of this diet, millions of people got their own copy of Dr. Atkins' New Diet Revolution to give it a try. The promise of quick weight loss without going through the usual low-calorie, low-fat, unpleasant diet that people trying to lose weight were used to, spawned extensive appeal. And that appeal would not have lasted through the years if it wasn't effective. This just goes to show that the Atkins Diet really works. How it works and how you can apply it to yourself is what this book is going to explain you. This book explains the basic principles of this diet, how you can make it effective for yourself, sample menu and recipes, together with other important things you need to know about this diet.

# Chapter 1: What is Atkins Diet?

The Atkins diet helps people in reducing their body fat and it also claims to increase the body's health. This can be attained by increasing the consumption of fats and meats, and decreasing carbohydrates and specific vegetables at the same time.

The Atkins diet aims to attain a considerable weight loss and offer a healthier lifestyle for the person trying to diet. Dr. Robert Atkins, its founder, believed that by increasing the number of fats and decreasing the consumption of carbohydrates, sugar, and salt, a person can significantly lose weight.

If you're planning to try out the Atkins diet, it's important that you know what's involved in trying to obtain the outcomes this diet claims to provide you. There are people that have misinterpreted what's involved with this diet and have successively suffered an opposing effect on their health. But what the Atkins diet claims to be could only be done if the person is entirely aware of this diet process. It is not like simply adding a fruit supplement to your diet and wait for the result! It means that you must clearly know that dietary supplements like minerals or vitamins and physical workout are essential to achieving the weight loss results.

When it comes to any diet plan, obeying the instructions is the key to controlling the weight successfully. Most of the time, people would think that indulging with little cravings like cookies wouldn't make a lot of difference. But adhering to a "no sweet rule" isn't only about losing weight, but it's also a test on your self-discipline. By going against these diet rules, you're also going against yourself at the same time.

By sticking closely to the diet rules, you are able to look ahead to some really remarkable, long-term results as long as you keep the proper nutrition that you need. It might also require checking the instructions of the diet regularly and making all essential changes.

# Chapter 2: How Does Atkins Diet Work?

This maybe one of the questions those people who are tired of dealing with the excess body fats keep asking all the time.

Atkins diet works by decreasing the consumption of foods that are rich in carbohydrates. As you lessen the carbohydrates consumption, your body burns stored fats. With this, the result significantly troubles the supply of insulin as a way of preventing the creation of fats within your system. When you make it a habit and your body starts to get used to this routine, you'll see that you won't crave for carbohydrates as you did before and this is where the idea of Atkins diet takes place.

The Atkins diet works in four different phases that you have to get used to attain the weight loss you want. These four phases are the induction phase, the ongoing weight loss, pre-maintenance stage, and the maintenance phase which we are going to discuss later on. All these phases are what establishes this diet and if you can follow and stick to this kind of diet, it is going to be easier for you to shed the weight you want to lose.

Dr. Atkins established the Atkins diet in 1972. His formula was:

Low carb = low insulin = ketosis phase = burning fat = losing weight

If a person lessens his consumption of carbohydrate to 30 to 40 grams per day, his body will get into a phase, which is known as ketosis. During ketosis phase, the body burns fat and it affects the insulin production in the liver. When you enter the phase of ketosis, the body will begin turning fat into fuel and your cravings for carbohydrates will lessen. The idea behind the Akins diet is that once you reduce your consumption of carbohydrate, your body will use the extra fat and you will start losing excess weight.

While other low carbohydrate diets make you count your carbohydrate consumption rather than calories, you're still depending on the fact that the calorie consumption will be lower than the usual. It's partially because of the fact that there are fewer calories in protein than in carbohydrate, and relatively due to the appetite restriction effects on the body.

You'll also see better outcomes if you pair this diet with a physical workout, because when the body is in a state of getting rid of fat rather than carbohydrates, clearly the more energy it uses, the more fat it burns.

# Chapter 3: The Four Phases of Atkins Diet Plan

As mentioned earlier, Atkins Diet plan includes four phases. The foods you eat should depend on the phase that you're in as well as on your metabolism level.

## Phase 1: The Induction Phase

This phase is clearly the most restraining and definitely, the most important phase of this diet because it's designed to help your body stop its cravings for carbohydrates. The carbohydrate consumption at the first stage is restricted to around 20 grams a day.

This first limit on the carbohydrate amount that you are primarily allowed to eat is what most people see as establishing the Atkins Diet. This, however, isn't the case, as other phases of this diet progressively let you increase your consumption level of carbohydrates.

The induction phase usually goes for about two weeks. If you stay within the carbohydrate food types that are allowed and calorie confines, you can eat as much as you want. However, you have to be careful because even though the Atkins Diet isn't a calorie-restricted diet, it will be a lot healthier to eat just healthy fats and protein.

Losing weight during the first phase is normally drastic because of many physiological effects of the diet. However, the weight loss that you experience at this phase is mostly body water loss because of the fact that the metabolism of glycogen for energy creates around 75% of water which is consequently passed out in the form of urine. That's why if you are following this diet, you are encouraged to drink plenty glasses of water mainly throughout this stage and also throughout the other phases of the program so as to avoid constipation and dehydration.

The main idea behind this difficult phase of the diet is to prepare your body for burning all the fat in the following phases. You are also going lose the most weight during this phase, making you persist with the diet until the end. In this phase you will have a list of foods you are allowed to eat with generous amounts of protein which include – but not limited to – the following:

- All types of fish
- All types poultry

- All shellfish (take note that mussels and oysters have higher level of carbohydrates, so it has to be limited to 4 ounces per day)

- All types of meat

- Eggs -Since eggs are an essential in the Atkins diet, and you can eat them more often. You can even get creative when preparing them, so it is less likely for you to get tired of eating them. Cooking them in different styles and adding healthy vegetables would be Atkins-friendly

- Cheese - Cheese has around 1 gram of carbohydrates per ounce, so consuming 3 to 4 ounces of cheese per day is the max at this phase of the diet

- Vegetables - Around 12 to 15 grams of your everyday carbohydrate consumption has to come from vegetables

- Beverages - When it comes to beverage, you can have club soda, caffeinated tea or coffee (1 to 2 cups a day), no-calorie seltzer water, bouillon, lime or lemon juice, water, herbal tea

Foods that you must avoid at all cost while at the Induction Phase:

- Grains and any food that are made with them, which include pastries, cake, bread, or anything else made with flour

- Any food that has extra sugars, which is the case with processed food

- Fruits and fruit juices

- Dairy products, apart from cheeses and cream in limited amounts

- Starchy vegetables like beets, potatoes, corn, etc.

- Legumes like peas and beans

- Deli salads, which normally contain extra sugars

- Alcoholic drinks

- Nuts, even though they're recommended after getting through the Induction Phase

## Phase 2:  Ongoing Weight Loss Phase or OWL Phase

The Ongoing Weight Loss phase of the diet is purposely aimed to slow the process of weight loss in order to establish the foundation for lasting weight loss management. The second phase also gives you the chance to start modifying the diet to suit your particular taste.

The second phase involves the slow addition of more nutrient dense carbohydrates into your regimen. But this slow addition is advised to primarily come from mostly vegetables like asparagus and cauliflower, then from other fiber rich and fresh nutrient sources.

Furthermore, you are not allowed to add over 5 grams of carbohydrate a week so as to define what the Atkins Diet calls the dieter's Critical Carbohydrate Level for Losing or CCLL – this being the everyday verge for carbohydrate intake. On condition that you continue to lose weight, you're allowed to increase your consumption of carbohydrate by 5 grams a week until the weight loss stalls, and then you go back to the prior carbohydrate intake level.

The Ongoing Weight Loss phase then lets you eat a wider variety of healthy foods which includes the ones you like most.

People who are following the Atkins Diet are encouraged to stick to the OWL phase until they have gotten to a stage where they are just around 5 to 10 pounds short of reaching their weight goal.

In this Phase, you gradually begin to add whole food carbs back to your diet, eating a minimum of 12 to 15 Net Carbs every day, and increasing the Net Carbs in 5-gram additions once a week or once or twice a month, whichever suits you best. There's no fixed amount on how long you should stick to the Phase 2 of the diet. The way this phase works is that you must use the phase 1 as your foundation.

## Phase 3: The Pre-Maintenance Phase

Atkins Diet's third phase is designed to prepare and inform you with the foretaste of what the proper eating habits you should have for a lifetime after finishing all the phases. This phase should be obligatory if you want to achieve permanent weight loss.

When you reach the 5 to 10 pounds goal weight of the second phase of the diet, you now would be required to get through the pre-maintenance phase in order to increase your day-to-day carbohydrate intake by 10 grams a week for as long as you carry on to lose weight. The idea is to carry on increasing the consumption of carbohydrate until you lose less than a pound every week.

When you reach your goal, you're then encouraged to stick to the same level upon which you reached your weight goal for another month or so before increasing your regular carbohydrate consumption by another 10 grams in order to see if you can carry on at that level without gaining any weight. You will continue making the 10 grams increase on a weekly basis for as long as you continue to lose weight regardless of how slow it may happen.

The extra carbohydrate food helps in providing better nutrition, diversity, and food enjoyment which makes it easier for you to follow the diet. This phase has to continue for at least 1 month but you're intensely encouraged to allow it to last for 2 or 3 months in order to attain the best results. The aim of this phase is to help you adopt the habits to be part of your permanent routine as you move to the fourth and last phase.

Lasting approximately 1 month, the third phase of the diet let you consume more carbohydrates in your diet, with 50 to 70 Net Carbs allowed every day. Now, you are only 10 pounds away from the weight you want to achieve, and you're adjusting your diet, precisely your personal carb balance for when you're done with this diet plan.

## Phase 4: The Lifetime Maintenance Phase

The last and fourth phase of the Atkins Diet is what we called the maintenance phase, which begins when the dieter has achieved his or her weight loss goal. The phase 4, you are allowed to make the most of a number of good carbohydrates you can eat from about 90 to 120 grams per day depending on the age, gender, and level of physical activity.

The Atkins Diet is therefore about preparing you to adjust to real-world challenges about efficiently losing and keeping healthy weight loss.

This Atkins Diet's 4-phase structure is therefore purposely intended to progressively help you to learn and adjust to a new healthy routine you need in order to keep the weight loss that this diet program has helped you achieve.

As effective as this diet plan seems to be, it gives you many options in terms of the foods you are allowed to consume. If the diet you choose includes a lot of sugars and bread, then you might have a hard time getting accustomed to your post-Atkins routine, but if you already have a nice healthy diet, the change to a low-carb diet should not be very hard. And even though it is, it is going to have a lot of benefits for your routine and weight, and following the Atkins should not be considered as a diet, but instead a change of lifestyle.

# Chapter 4: Atkins Diet Sample Meal Plan

Atkins diet meals include five meals a day. Every dish could be very healthy and interesting to everyone regardless of what their tastes are. The five meals include the breakfast, morning tea, lunch, afternoon tea, and of course, the dinner. On top of five meals per day, this diet also includes four phases which were mentioned in the previous chapter. In order to help you on planning your meal while you are on the diet, here is a sample menu of what you can eat while you are on the diet:

## Phase 1

The phase one normally lasts for two weeks and restricts you to 12 to 15 grams of carbohydrates a day.

### BREAKFAST

### Sausage Zucchini Frittata

### Ingredients:
- 1/3 cup heavy cream
- 1 cup shredded sharp cheddar cheese
- 1 cup shredded mozzarella cheese
- 1 teaspoon of Italian seasoning

- 1 teaspoon of minced basil
- 2 sliced scallions
- 2 cups of unpeeled shredded zucchini
- 4 eggs
- 4 oz. of cubed cream cheese
- 8 oz. of sliced sausage

## Instructions:

1. Preheat the oven to 325°F. Spray 8-inch pie pan with cooking spray. Drain the sliced sausage well, place on the bottom of the pan. Top with scallions, zucchini, and the seasonings.

2. Whisk eggs and add cream, then slowly pour in the sausage mixture. Add the cubed cream cheese on top, then the cheddar and mozzarella. Bake for 45 minutes or the middle comes out clean when you poke it with a knife. Serve and enjoy.

Per serving: 4g carbs; 1g fiber; 18g protein; 38g fat; 435 calories

## Happy Breakfast Meatballs

## Ingredients:

- ½ pounds shredded cheddar cheese
- 1 pound ground beef
- 2 tablespoon of instant minced onion

- 2 pounds of sausage
- 3 large eggs
- black pepper to taste

## Instruction:

1. Preheat the oven to 350°F. Put all ingredients together and mix thoroughly.
2. Roll into 1 ½ inch balls and put on cookie sheet. Bake for about 20 to 25 minutes.

Per serving: 87 calories; 0.137 carbohydrates; 5.36 proteins


## Breakfast Quiche Lorraine

## Ingredients:

- 1 cup of Half and Half
- 1 cup of whipping cream
- 1 cup Swiss cheese
- 4 large beaten eggs
- 9 slices of crumbled bacon
- Salt and Pepper to taste
- Dash of nutmeg

## Instructions:

1. Combine all together and pour into a pie dish
2. Bake at 400°F for about 45 to 50 minutes or until the pick comes out clean.

Per serving: 1929 calories; 170g fat; 24g carbs; 79g protein

# LUNCH / DINNER

## Herb-Butter Blended Baked Fish

### Ingredients:
- 1 serving of Herb-Butter Blend
- 1 cup of floweret Broccoli Flower Clusters
- 6 ounces of farmed catfish

### Instructions:
1. Preheat the oven to 350°F.
2. Lay the fish on a square piece of foil. Drizzle the fish with salt and ground pepper to taste. Place the broccoli florets all over the fish.
3. Fold in the sides of the foil and fold tightly in order to create a sealed sachet.
4. Bake for 10 to 15 minutes until the fish is peeling and broccoli becomes tender.
5. Put the fish on a plate, open the foil and put Herb-Butter Blend all over and serve.

Per serving: 28.7g protein; 25.9g fat; 2.2g fiber; 362 calories

## Atkins Beef Burger

### Ingredients:
- ¼ cup of sliced tomatoes
- ¼ cup smashed feta cheese

- ½ teaspoon of salt
- ½ teaspoon of black pepper
- ½ cup of baby spinach
- 1 scallions
- 1 pound ground beef
- 1 ½ teaspoons of fresh dill

**Instructions:**

1. Combine ground beef, spinach, scallion, tomato, fresh dill, feta, salt and pepper together. Form the mixture into patties.
2. Fry or grill over medium-high heat for about 5 minutes on each side or until it gets brown.

Per serving: 24.3g protein; 13.4g fat; 0.5g fiber; 231 calories

## Cauliflower Risotto

**Ingredients:**

- ½ cup bouillon vegetable broth
- ½ cup of grated parmesan cheese
- 1 tablespoon of chopped shallots
- 1 tablespoon of extra virgin olive oil
- 2 tablespoons of heavy cream
- 2 cups cauliflower
- 2 tablespoons parsley

**Instructions:**

1. Place the cauliflower florets in a blender or food processor and pulse until they're the size of grains of rice.
2. Place the pan over medium heat and cook the shallots in the olive oil until it becomes tender.
3. Add in the cauliflower; fold in the vegetable stock and cook for about 10 minutes or until it becomes tender.
4. Add in the cream, cheese, and parsley.
5. Add salt and pepper to taste.

Per serving: 5.1g protein; 9.3g fat; 1.3g fiber; 117 calories

## SNACK

### Cheesy Asparagus Rolls

**Ingredients:**

- 6 slices of Smart Deli Roast Turkey Style
- 3 spears of Asparagus
- 1 ounce of sliced Swiss cheese

**Instructions:**

1. Place 2 slices of turkey and then put on a slice of Swiss cheese.

2. Put 1 asparagus spear at one end and then roll over. Pin a toothpick at the center to keep the roll from unraveling. Serve.

Per serving: 28.3g protein; 13.1g fat; 4.2g fiber; 270 calories

# Grilled Cheese with Fresh Tomato

## Ingredients:
- ¼ cup of shredded cheddar cheese
- 1 serving Atkins cloud bread
- 1 teaspoon unsalted butter stick
- 2 slices of tomatoes

## Instructions:
1. Preheat the pan over medium-high heat. Put the butter and let it melt.
2. Slice a piece of bread into two thinner slices and put them in the pan. Brown both sides; add the cheese over a slice of bread while browning the other side.
3. Put two slices of tomato on the melted cheese, dash of salt and black pepper, and then out the other piece over the top of the bread.

Per serving: 25.2g protein; 37.3g fat; 0.5g fiber; 450 calories

## Crispy Zucchini Delight

## Ingredients:
- ¼ teaspoon black pepper
- ¼ teaspoon salt
- 2 medium zucchinis
- 2 tablespoons grated parmesan cheese
- 2 tablespoons of extra virgin olive oil

## Instructions:

1. Cut the zucchini into ¼ inch slices. Cover both sides with extra-virgin olive oil and dash with salt, pepper, and parmesan.

2. Place on a baking sheet in one layer and bake in a 400°F oven for about 10 minutes.

Per serving: 2.2g protein; 8g fat; 0.9g fiber; 88 calories

# Phase Two

The phase two lets you add more foods back into your regular diet and up to 25 grams of carbohydrates every day.

## Breakfast

## Coconut and Almond Muffin

## Ingredients:

- 1/8 cup Almond Meal Flour
- 1/3 tbsp Organic High Fiber Coconut Flour
- 1 tsp Sucralose Based Sweetener (Sugar Substitute)
- 1/2 tsp Cinnamon
- 1/4 tsp Baking Powder (Straight Phosphate, Double Acting)
- 1/8 tsp Salt

- 1 large Egg (Whole)
- 1/3 tbsp Extra Virgin Olive Oil

## Directions:

1. Add all of the dry ingredients in a coffee mug. Mix well to combine.
2. Mix in the egg and oil.
3. Place in the microwave for 60 seconds. Remove or eat from the mug.

Per serving: 9.7g protein; 16.8g fat; 3g fiber; 207 calories

## Blueberry Almond Pancakes

## Ingredients:

- 1/16 cup of blanched almond flour
- 1/8 cup of dry whole grain soy flour
- ¼ teaspoon baking powder
- ¼ cup chopped blueberries
- ½ ounce curd creamed cottage cheese
- 1 large egg
- 2 tablespoons of vanilla whey protein

## Instructions:

1. Mix the almond flour, soy flour, protein powder, chopped blueberries, and baking powder altogether. Add the beaten egg and cheese until fully combined.

2. Heat a pan on medium heat. Grease in lightly with canola oil or butter.

3. Using about ¼ cup per pancake, place the batter on the pan. When bubbles start to form in the middle of every pancake, flip over and cook until it becomes firm.

Per serving: 20.3g Protein; 10g Fat; 2.5g Fiber; 212 Calories

## Mexican Peppers Bombs

### Ingredients:

- ¼ of cup shredded cheddar cheese
- ½ cup of chopped onions
- 2 sweet red peppers
- 3 large eggs
- 4 ounces ground beef
- 4 ounces pork and beef chorizo

### Directions:

1. Preheat the oven to 400°F. Place a baking sheet on a foil.

2. Cook the chorizo, stir will split up the lumps, until browned.

3. Put the ground beef and chorizo in a large bowl and mix with the cheese, onion, and eggs.

4. Cut the peppers in half lengthways. Take out the seeds as well as the ribs.

5. Fill every pepper with a quarter of the mixture. Add the prepared baking sheet. Bake for 25 to30 minutes, serve and enjoy.

Per serving: 21.3g Protein; 20.1g Fat; 1.5g Fiber; 298 Calories

## LUNCH/DINNER

### Spiced Bacon Asparagus Rolls

### Ingredients:

- ½ teaspoon of sucralose-based sweetener
- 1 teaspoon of chili powder
- 4 slices bacon
- 24 spears asparagus

### Instructions:

1. Infuse toothpicks in warm water for about 15-20 minutes.

2. Preheat the grill. Place a sheet of wax paper on a pan and put to one side. Put the chili powder and sucralose in a bowl.

3. Cut the bacon into strips. Place them on a pan and drizzle with the mixture of chili powder.

4. Cover three asparagus spears alongside a slice of bacon; secure both ends using a toothpick.

5. Grill the rolls on medium-low heat for about 10 minutes or until bacon becomes crispy.

6. Remove the toothpicks and serve.

Per serving: 5g protein; 10.2g fat; 2.4g fiber; 128 calories

## Juicy Baked Meatballs

## Ingredients:

- ¼ teaspoon black pepper
- ½ pound ground veal
- ½ large scallions
- ½ pound ground beef
- ½ pound ground pork
- ½ teaspoon salt
- ½ cup of grated parmesan cheese
- 1 tablespoon extra-virgin olive oil
- 1 ½ tablespoons garlic
- 2 eggs

## Ingredients:

1. Heat the oven to 375°F.

2. In a pan, set on high heat, cook the onion for 5 minutes; stir frequently until it becomes soft. Add the minced garlic and cook another minute.

3. Put it in a bowl and add ground meats, eggs, cheese, salt, and pepper. Roll into balls. Put on a roll pan.

4. Bake for about 20 to 25 minutes until the layer gets brown.

Per serving: 38.6g protein; 26.7g fat; 0.2g fiber; 409 calories

## Beef Tenderloin

### Ingredients:

- ½ teaspoon of black pepper
- 1 teaspoon salt
- 1 ½ tablespoons of extra virgin olive oil
- 4 pounds of beef tenderloin

### Instructions:

1. Heat the oven to 425°F.

2. Put the beef in a roll pan. Cover with oil, pepper, and salt. Put a meat thermometer. Roast for about 30 to 35 minutes to attain medium-rare doneness. The thermometer has to show 125°F.

3. Place on a cutting board; cover with foil and let rest for about 10 minutes before serving.

Per serving: 44.5g protein; 43.8g fat 0g; fiber; 583 calories

## SNACK

### Chili Roasted Nut

**Ingredients:**
- 1 teaspoon salt
- 1 teaspoon canola vegetable oil
- 1 ½ tablespoons chili powder
- 2 cup macadamia nuts

**Instructions:**
1. Heat the oven to 300°F.
2. Place the nuts covered with oil over a sheet pan and bake for about 25 to 30 minutes, until it turns golden.
3. Put in a bowl; drizzle with chili powder and salt.

Per serving: 3.5g Protein; 34.6g Fat; 3.8g Fiber; 328 Calories

### Fresh Berry Tarts with Cream

**Ingredients:**
- ¼ cup heavy cream
- ½ cup blueberries
- ½ cup raspberries
- 2/3 cup of almonds
- 2 tablespoons of sucralose-based sweetener

**Instructions:**

1. Heat the broiler. Chop the almonds and divide them into four ramekins. Sprinkle the almonds with sucralose based sweetener. Put the ramekins on a baking sheet and broil until the layer of the nuts get golden and the sucralose-based sweetener has melted. Take off and let it cool down at the room temperature.

2. Put the heavy cream and remaining sucralose based sweetener until the volume doubles up. Put a quarter of blueberries and a quarter of raspberries in every ramekin and top with a spoonful of whipped cream.

Per serving: 4.5g protein; 14.6g fat; 3.6g fiber; 177 calories

## Ham Covered Asparagus Rolls

**Ingredients:**

- 2 tablespoons real mayonnaise
- 2 slices of muenster cheese
- 4 ounces fresh ham
- 4 spears of asparagus

**Instructions:**

1. Slice the ham and Muenster into four thin slices.

2. Layer ham with cheese and mayonnaise. Roll them over the asparagus and cheese stick. Dip them into the mayonnaise.

Per serving: 35.1g protein; 43.1g fat; 1.6g fiber; 546 calories

# PHASE THREE

In phase three, you have to continue adding carbohydrates back to your everyday diet. The difference is that you have to choose a number of carbohydrates you consume on a daily basis. It is recommended to add 10 grams of carbohydrates every week, but as long as you are losing weight, then you are doing the right thing.

## Breakfast

Cheesy Mushroom Omelet

### Ingredients:
- ¼ cup of cheddar cheese
- ¼ cup of shiitake mushrooms
- 1/3 cup of onions
- 1 teaspoon of canola vegetable oil
- 2 eggs

### Instructions:
1. Heat oil in a pan over medium-high heat. Add the mushrooms and onion slices. Cook for approximately 5 minutes until the onions get translucent and mushrooms get soft. Take it off from pan and set aside.
2. Add the eggs to the pan. Cook for about 3 minutes. Turn over and cook another 2 to 3 minutes.

3. Add the mushrooms and onion to half of omelet and put cheese on top. Fold the half and cook for 1 to 2 minutes more until the cheese melts.

Per serving: 21.5g Protein; 23.9g Fat; 2.3g Fiber; 339 Calories

## Creamy Atkins Waffles

## Ingredients:
- ¼ teaspoon salt
- 1 individual packet sucralose based sweetener
- 1 cup cream
- 1 egg
- 2 teaspoons of baking powder

## Instructions:
1. In a big bowl, mix together a cup of baking mix, sucralose based sweetener, baking powder, and salt.
2. In a separate large bowl, combine the cream and egg.
3. Add the dry ingredients to the wet ingredients and mix thoroughly until there won't be any lumps.
4. Set aside the mixture sit for about 5 minutes.
5. Heat the waffle iron and slowly pour in the batter.
6. Close the waffle iron and let it cook for about 1 to 2 minutes or until it turns golden red.

Per serving: 21.4g protein; 9g fat; 1.9g fiber; 193 calories

## Corned Beef Hash Brown

### Ingredients:

- ½ cup heavy cream
- ½ cup chopped onions
- 2 cups turnips
- 3 tablespoons canola vegetable oil
- 16 ounces corned beef brisket

### Instructions:

1. Toss cubed beef and turnips together in a bowl. Add onion and heavy cream and stir to combine.
2. Heat the oil in a nonstick pan over medium-low heat for about a minute. Add the beef mixture and cook for about 10 minutes or until you form a crust.
3. Turn the hash to cook the other side.

Per serving: 22g Protein; 43.2g Fat; 1.9g Fiber; 506 Calories

## LUNCH/DINNER

## Oriental Vegetable Bowl

### Ingredients:

- ½ ounces cilantro
- 1 carrot
- 1 garlic clove
- 1 cup chopped red tomatoes

- 1 pepper Serrano pepper
- 2 cups of mushroom pieces
- 2 cups shredded Chinese cabbage
- 3 teaspoons ginger
- 3 cups of chopped spring onions
- 4 tablespoons tamari soybean sauce
- 6 cups chicken broth
- 6 ounces of firm silken tofu

## Instructions:

1. Boil broth and tamari soybean sauce in a saucepan.
2. When it boils, reduce the heat and add the Chinese cabbage, mushrooms, minced garlic, ginger, and chili. Let it simmer for 5 minutes, until the cabbage is tender.
3. Add green onions, tomatoes, carrot, and tofu.
4. Transfer to a bowl and serve with spring onion on top.

Per serving: 6.7g Protein; 2.1g Fat; 1.8g Fiber; 65 Calories

## Asian Coleslaw Delight

## Ingredients:

- 1 large carrots
- 1 teaspoon sucralose based sweetener
- 1 tablespoon toasted sesame oil
- 1 cup chopped snow peas
- 1 tablespoon tamari soybean sauce
- 2 tablespoons extra virgin olive oil

- 2 tablespoons sodium and sugar-free rice vinegar
- 2 teaspoons ginger
- 12 ounces Chinese cabbage

## Instructions:

1. Put the cabbage in a bowl; grate the carrot into the cabbage. Add in the snow peas.
2. In a separate bowl, combine vinegar, oils, ginger, tamari, and sugar substitute.
3. Add the dressing on the salad; combine to coat. Add salt to taste.

Per serving: 1.7g Protein; 7g Fat; 1.4g Fiber; 82 Calories


## Bacon-Egg Salad Flat-Out Roll

## Ingredients:

- ½ teaspoon yellow mustard
- 1 flatbread light original flatbread
- 1 tablespoons mayonnaise
- 1 ½ ounces cooked turkey bacon
- 2 boiled eggs

## Instructions:

1. Combine the chopped eggs, mustard, and mayonnaise. Add pepper and salt to taste.
2. Spread the mixture around the flat-out. Put some cooked crumbled bacon on top.
3. Roll and serve.

Per serving 34.4g Protein; 36.1g Fat; 10.2g Fiber; 511 Calories

## SNACK

### Avocado Salsa

### Ingredients:

- 1/8 cup cilantro
- 1/8 teaspoon black pepper
- 1/8 teaspoon salt
- ½ jalapeño peppers
- 1 avocados
- 1 red tomato
- 1 red onion
- 2 tablespoons lime juice

### Instructions:

1. Chop the onion, tomato, and jalapeño.
2. Mix the avocado, jalapeño, onion, and lime juice gently. Don't mash.
3. Add cilantro and tomato and drizzle salt and pepper to taste.
4. Cover and chill for at least 2 hours before serving.

Per serving: 1.1g Protein; 5.3g Fat; 3g Fiber; 71 Calories

## Fresh Caprese Salad

### Ingredients:

- 1 tablespoon basil
- 1 tablespoon extra-virgin olive oil
- 2 ounces fresh mozzarella
- 5 cherries cherry tomatoes

### Instructions:

1. Slice the mozzarella and tomatoes.
2. Drizzle with extra-virgin olive oil.
3. Add the fresh chopped basil leaves over the salad. Serve immediately.

Per serving: 10.1g Protein; 27.4g Fat; 1.1g Fiber; 294 Calories

## Yummy Hummus on Cucumber

### Ingredients:

- 1 cup slice of peeled Cucumber
- 4 tablespoons Organic Hummus Classic

### Instructions:

1. Slice the cucumber and put a spoonful of hummus on top. Enjoy.

Per serving: 5.4g Protein; 5.9g Fat; 4.1g Fiber; 115 Calories

# Phase Four

The meals you eat in the maintenance phase should contain anywhere from 10 to 20 grams of carbohydrates, so you could easily choose from a wider food variety.

**BREAKFAST**

**Cheesy Onion Omelet**

**Ingredients:**
- ½ cup cheddar cheese
- 1/3 cup cut onions
- 1 tablespoon olive oil
- 2 eggs

**Instruction:**
1. Cook white onions in a tablespoon of olive oil in a pan over medium heat until it becomes tender and translucent. Transfer to a plate and set aside.
2. Lightly beat the eggs and cook it in the same pan. Cook until bubbles are formed and carefully turn over. Put some onions and cheese on the half surface. Cook for another minute, fold other on the side and add cheese and onions again. Cook for another minute.
3. Transfer the omelet to a plate and add salt and pepper to taste.

Per serving: 26.7g Protein; 41.8g Fat; 0.9g Fiber; 509 Calories

## Cheesy Bell Pepper Rings

### Ingredients:

- ¼ cup shredded mozzarella cheese
- ¼ apple
- ¼ banana
- ¼ cup raspberries
- ½ sweet red pepper
- ½ fruit kiwi fruit
- 1 teaspoon olive oil
- 2 eggs

### Instructions:

1. Slice the bell pepper to form two 1-inch rings.
2. Heat nonstick pan with some olive oil on medium high heat.
3. Crack 1 egg inside the bell pepper ring, cook for about 2 minutes then add 2 tablespoons of water on the pan to steam the pepper and egg for another 3 to 5 minutes until the egg is cooked.
4. Put cheese on top. Cover the pan for at least 1 minute to melt the cheese.
5. On a separate bowl, combine the fruits and serve together with the pepper rings.

Per serving: 19.9g Protein; 20.6g Fat; 5.8g Fiber; 361 Calories

# Scrambled Egg with Spinach and Feta

## Ingredients:

- ½ ounce feta cheese
- 1 tablespoons canola vegetable oil
- 2 eggs
- 2 1/16 cups baby spinach

## Instructions:

1. In a nonstick pan, wilt the spinach with a tablespoon of water on medium heat.
2. Add beaten eggs and cheese and cook until it's cooked.
3. Drizzle with salt and black pepper, serve and enjoy.

Per serving: 16.9g Protein; 27.7g Fat; 1.3g Fiber; 330 Calories

## LUNCH/DINNER

## Nutty Arugula Salad

## Ingredients:

- ½ cup crumbled gorgonzola cheese
- 1 medium pear
- 2 servings of maple-Dijon vinaigrette
- 10 ounces arugula
- 40 hazelnuts

## Instructions:

1. Toast the hazelnuts in a pan for approximately 15 minutes; let it cool down and rub off on the surface gently, chop, and set aside.

2. Add the Maple-Dijon Vinaigrette with the arugula and cheese. Put onto serving plates.

3. Arrange the pear slices and drizzle with hazelnuts.

Per serving: 7.1g Protein; 20g Fat; 4.4g Fiber; 244 Calories

## Chili Cheesy Chops

### Ingredients:

- 1/3 cup cheddar cheese
- 1 tablespoon canola vegetable oil
- 1 teaspoon cumin
- 2 ounces salsa
- 2 tablespoons cream cheese
- 2 ¼ ounces green chili peppers
- 14 ounces pork chops or roasts

### Instructions:

1. Heat oil in a pan over medium-high heat. Season chops with some pepper and salt. Brown chops for about 2 minutes for every side.

2. Combine chilies, cumin, and salsa in a bowl. Put the mixture on the chops. Reduce the heat to low, put the

cover on the pan, and simmer chops for about 5 minutes or until it's cooked.

3.  Combine the cheeses in a bowl. Split cheese mixture on the chops, cover, and cook for a minute to melt the cheese.

Per serving: 44g protein; 30.1g fat; 1.4g fiber; 481 calories

## Baked Meatballs

### Ingredients:

- ¼ teaspoon black pepper
- ½ pound ground veal
- ½ pound ground pork
- ½ pound ground beef
- ½ teaspoon salt
- ½ cup parmesan cheese
- ½ spring onion
- 1 tablespoon extra-virgin olive oil
- 1 ½ tablespoons garlic
- 2 eggs

### Instructions:

1.  Preheat the oven to 375°F.
2.  In a pan, heat the oil and cook the onion for 5 minutes until it softened. Add the minced garlic and cook for another minute.

3. Put to a bowl and combine with ground meats, eggs, cheese, pepper, and salt. Roll the mixture into balls. Put on a pan.

4. Bake for about 20 to 25 minutes, or until they're browned.

Per serving: 38.6g Protein; 26.7g Fat; 0.2g Fiber; 409 Calories

**SNACK**

## Atkins Advantage Peanut Butter Granola Bar with Creamy Strawberries

### Ingredients:

- ½ cup Greek yogurt
- 1 serving Atkins Advantage Peanut Butter Granola Bar
- 5 large strawberries

### Instructions:

1. In a parfait glass, put the chopped granola bar in a layer with the strawberries and yogurt.

Per serving: 24.1g Protein; 9.5g Fat; 6.8g Fiber; 314 Calories

## Healthy Blackberry Smoothie

### Ingredients:

- 1/16 cup flaxseed meal
- 1/16 teaspoon allspice ground

- ¼ cup frozen blackberries
- ¼ teaspoon cinnamon
- ½ teaspoon vanilla extract
- 1 cup unsweetened coconut milk
- 1 scoop vanilla whey protein

## Instructions:

1. Mix the frozen blackberries, coconut milk, vanilla, protein powder, and spices using a blender. Blend until smooth.

Per serving: 21.8g Protein; 9.8g Fat; 5.8g Fiber; 221 Calories

## Black Olives with Cheddar

## Ingredients:

- 1 ounce of Cheddar Cheese
- 7 Greek olives Black Olives

## Instructions:

1. Cube the cheese and put a hole in the olive with a toothpick.
2. Eat and enjoy.

Per serving: 7.3g Protein; 12.7g Fat; 1g Fiber; 150 Calories

# Chapter 5: Substitute for Carbohydrates

Sugar substitutes are becoming more and more popular. Everyone has different thoughts about artificial sweeteners like Splenda and Aspartame. These substitutes can be really helpful in preparing low-carbohydrate food without consuming sugar. But many people think that artificial sweeteners can actually make them crave more. If you're having this problem, then it's advisable to remove them completely from your regimen.

Bread is a big challenge for people going through Atkins diet. Bread is widely eaten anywhere, and removing it from your diet can be a bit difficult. But luckily, there are some low-carbohydrate bread you can buy in the market, but you need to pay attention to hidden carbohydrates and other unacceptable ingredients it may include.

A lot of people love pasta, but eating it plain wouldn't be much enjoyable. The topping is what makes the pasta desirable. A simple solution to avoid the high carbohydrates from pasta is to take the toppings and place them on to something else. Spaghetti squash or zucchini are a good replacement for pasta.

Another high carbohydrate food that is difficult to avoid is rice. The popular replacement for this is cauliflower. Cauliflower is also a good substitute for potatoes.

Pizza could be alternatively home-produced. You are able to make little pizzas with low-carbohydrate tortillas as your crust. Alternatively, you are able to use big Portobello mushrooms.

These substitutes are good in helping you satisfy your cravings. Give them a try and you will see that they are as enjoyable as your old favorites.

# Conclusion

The Atkins Diet had faced bad image in the past years, mostly because some people believe that it is not healthy. In fact, whilst it's a fairly radical change in diet which changes a person's metabolism, it is not that bad. A lot of people who criticize this diet have no idea how this diet works.

A lot of people believe that eating fatty food is bad for the health. Generally, it can be, however, the Atkins Diet uses fat in a different way. It can burn more fat. So the increased consumption of fat actually helps you to make the diet work.

It's also a fact that once you begin eating normal carbohydrates again, you will gain the weight back. However, the Atkins Diet teaches you to differentiate the bad carbohydrates from the good ones. It teaches you how to lessen the consumption of carbohydrate to help you lose weight. Basically, this diet plan is a lifestyle you have to apply to your life, so of course, if you would like to begin eating cake again on a daily basis, it's up to you, but expect your weight to go back again. The idea of this diet is that it's a low-carb diet that does not include normal consumption of carbohydrate.

There are a lot of success stories provided by people who tried this diet, and a lot of people who have lost their weight. So, if you want to find an easier way to follow the diet plan and something you can easily maintain, then Atkins Diet is worth a try.

www.ingramcontent.com/pod-product-compliance
Lightning Source LLC
Chambersburg PA
CBHW071257280526
45788CB00004B/1741